Ultimate Sugar Addiction Detox Guide!

Sugar Addiction

How To Beat Cravings Naturally And Cure Sugar Addiction With This Ultimate Sugar Detox Diet Formula!

Sarah Brooks

STOP!!! Before you read any further....Would you like to know the Secrets of Body Transformation?

If your answer is yes, then you are not alone. Thousands of people are looking for the secret to rapidly burn body fat, keep the weight off, become healthier, and truly transform their body and life for good.

If you have been searching for these answers without much luck, you are in the right place!

Not only will you gain incredible insight in this book, but because I want to make sure to give you as much value as possible, right now for a limited time you can get full **100% FREE access to a VIP bonus EBook** entitled **THE 7 KEYS TO BODY TRANSFORMATION!**

Just Go Here For Free Instant Access:

www.liveFitVIP.com

Table Of Contents

Introduction

I want to thank you and congratulate you for purchasing the book, ULTIMATE SUGAR ADDICTION DETOX GUIDE: How To Beat Cravings Naturally and Cure Sugar Addiction With This Ultimate Sugar Detox Diet Formula!

This "Sugar Addiction" book contains proven steps and strategies on how to naturally curb your sugar cravings and eventually free you from sugar addiction.

All forms of addiction are naturally rewarding, and it is no different with sugar. Though it is neither drug nor alcohol, the effects of sugar addiction can be detrimental to health and behavior.

It is important that you recognize if you are addicted to sugar so that you can avoid the potentially harmful effects of this addiction. The book highlights signs and symptoms of sugar addiction and natural means to beat it. It will help you realize the possible consequences of not addressing and bringing to an end this addiction.

You will also find helpful sugar detox diet recipes, recipes for smoothies, herbal remedies and natural ingredients that curb sugar cravings.

Thanks again for purchasing this book, I hope you enjoy it!

Chapter 1: Introduction For Sugar Addiction

Addiction is a condition of habitual engagement in something that is naturally rewarding. The usual addictions that people hear about involve alcohol, tobacco, and illegal drugs, but there are also potential non-drug compulsive indulgences that enslave people. These include addictions to food, gambling, computers, sex and exercise.

Addiction is often attributed to behavioral problems. However, some addictions blame genetics as the root cause. Addiction means one is preoccupied with substance and continues to use it despite undesirable consequences, is always in denial and has impaired management over his behavior over the element of addiction. Most addictions are characterized by instantaneous gratification and harmful, and sometimes fatal, effects.

No one is immune to addiction: it can afflict anyone from anywhere. One has to realize that every form of addiction is bad, regardless of the substance, idealism or behavior. Even the simplest substance that we use in everyday life can be a cause of addiction if we do not exercise control over our habits and patterns.

Take sugar, for example. That simple stuff is just so enjoyable and it makes you feel so good. The more sweets you have, the more you want. Moreover, it is so hard to keep away from it because it is already part of your everyday life.

Sugar is in no way illegal or dangerous. It is a harmless substance and is essentially useful. However, everything should be taken in moderation. Studies have shown that sugar can be as addictive and as intoxicating as alcohol, and like other things taken in excess, it can cause problems.

Sugar addiction can lead to weight gain, heart diseases, binge eating and cravings. In addition to shaking the body's homeostasis, there is a host of other consequences that you have to deal with if you are addicted to sugar:

- Sugar can slightly impair your immune system and weaken your defenses against infectious disease.
- Sugar interferes with the absorption of certain minerals in your body such as calcium and magnesium
- Sugar is detrimental to behavior in that it causes a rush of adrenaline, stimulates hyperactivity and anxiety, causes difficulty in concentration and even induces crankiness.
- Sugar may generate a considerable increase in total cholesterol, in triglycerides and other bad cholesterol while decreasing good cholesterol.
- Sugar can boost systolic blood pressure.
- Sugar feeds cancer cells and cause the development of certain cancers, such as that of the prostate, breast, ovaries, pancreas, rectum, gallbladder, lung, and stomach.
- Sugar can cause hypoglycemia.
- Sugar can deteriorate the eyesight.
- Sugar can cause gastrointestinal tract problems such as indigestion, malabsorption and acidic digestive tracts and increase the risk of Crohn's disease and ulcers.
- Sugar can trigger premature aging.
- Sugar can cause tooth decay, gum disease and other periodontal diseases.
- Sugar contributes to obesity.
- Sugar can result in asthma, arthritis, multiple sclerosis and other autoimmune diseases.
- Sugar can cause gallstones, appendicitis, varicose veins and can contribute to osteoporosis.
- Sugar can lead to diabetes.
- Sugar can cause migraines and headaches.
- Sugar can cause learning disorders by reducing learning capacity.
- Sugar can increase your risk of Alzheimer's disease.
-

Sugar comes into our body through our consumption of regular food like carbohydrates. Some sugars move stealthily into our system through unnoticeable stuff like catsup and teriyaki sauce. The more obvious sources are cookies, ice cream, cakes and other candies. Since even healthy yoghurt has sugar, we find that we aren't safe from sugar and its potential effects.

Sugar consumption should be limited to seven percent (7%) or less of daily intake of calorie. This roughly accounts for 100 calories or an equivalent of six (6) to nine (9) teaspoons of sugar. To put things in perspective, the amount of sugar in one glazed doughnut is equivalent to 6 teaspoons and a regular can of soda, which is 12-ounces, contains 8-10 teaspoons of sugar.

Sugar intake releases good hormones called serotonin which gives the body a feeling of euphoria. However this rush of hormone is only temporary and your body soon starts to crash and feel tired and lethargic. Sugar rush is not always good.

The more sugar intake you have, the more tolerance your body develops. This means that sugar addiction is due to food choices and dietary habits. Your intense craving for sugar is not hereditary. This also means that you can cut out on sugar and free yourself from addiction.

Chapter 2: Signs That You May Be Addicted To Sugar

Addiction, as mentioned in the first chapter, is the persistent and compulsive use or intake of a known harmful substance. Addiction to sugar can be such a case. People who insist on consuming sugar in large amounts despite the adverse consequences attached to it and can't seem to stop are addicted to sugar.

Simply liking ice cream and cakes does not necessarily equate to sugar addiction, but how do you know if it is too much? Here are signs and symptoms that you can check to see if you are addicted to sugar.

1. *Consistent sugar cravings at regular times each day.*
    Do you find yourself wanting to eat something sweet after dinner or lunch? If you always have sugar cravings at the same time every day, it is possible that you are highly dependent on sugar to give you an energy boost at these specific times, or simply to feel good.

2. *You have an all-day long craving for sugar.*
    Do you think about sweets the whole day? Drink a lot of fruit juice or soda, take your coffee extra sweet or chew on a cookie any time of the day? Then your craving may be stronger than just the need for an energy or emotional boost. If you find yourself spontaneously indulging in something sweet all day, then you are sugar dependent.

3. *You have a persistent sweet tooth*
    When you find that you cannot avoid not having dessert after meals, it is probably more than just liking sweets. Addiction means you have a compulsive desire to have something and cannot turn it down.

4. *You are uncomfortable when you try to cut back*

Do you feel irritable when you think about reducing your sugar intake? Do you experience withdrawal symptoms such as headaches, nausea, fatigue, moodiness and anxiety when you cut back? Then you are addicted to sugar.

If you are addicted to sugar, do not fret. You can be free from this addiction and live a healthier life. Do not worry about suffering uncomfortable symptoms when you withdraw from sweets. It may be a roller coaster ride but if you continue on your journey to being sugar-free, you will find that these symptoms will fade.

Chapter 3: Types Of Sugar Addiction And How To Beat Cravings Naturally

The human body cannot handle a sugar overload hence the many cases of diabetes, cancer and heart diseases. However, even if doctors tell the people to cut back on sugar, they find that it takes up a third of our daily caloric intake. This is because sugar is highly addictive and leads to loss of control and subsequent cravings.

As you tolerate sugar in your body, the body increases its threshold and you will find that you need more sugar the deeper you get into the addiction. There are four types of sugar addiction: thyroid failure, yeast infection, adrenaline overload and menopause or PMT.

Here are the signs you can check to see which sugar addiction you have which makes you crave and tolerate sugar in your body. The good news is that you can reverse the tolerance and reduce your sugar intake naturally.

- *Thyroid failure*

  Signs of thyroid failure include being stressed all the time, feeling tired or fatigued and craving sweets throughout the day. You may have an underactive thyroid gland that gives that feeling of fatigue. Likewise, you feel tension or stress in your muscles when they do not get enough energy needed to function because of the underactive thyroid gland. Frequent headaches caused by muscle tension are also signs of thyroid failure.

  To ease this problem, you need to drink more water. Hydrating your body will result in flushing your system effectively. You also need to cut back on your caffeine intake as well as processed foods. Switching to herbal tea drinks and whole foods will keep your blood sugar levels stable. When you don't get enough rest and are tired, your body turns to sugar for artificial energy which eventually leads to addiction. Curb that by getting enough rest. Sleeping more will mean more energy for you, thereby reducing your appetite and sugar cravings.

- *Yeast infection*

When you find that you cannot go through the day without any bread or a dose of sugar, then you possibly have yeast infection. Yeast infection may be due to a growth of bad bacteria in your body, usually the result of having to take a lot of antacids or antibiotics. The gut has good bacteria that may be killed by antibiotics. Antacids, on the other hand, neutralize the acid in the stomach that deals with the bad bacteria.

Yeast feeds on sugar and triggers your body's craving for sugar. Bread and sweets easily convert to glucose that's why you find the constant need to eat them. However, the more you take sugar in, the more the yeast will multiply, and the more your cravings will intensify; a deadly cycle that you need to stop.

First, you can take in probiotics and yoghurt to help the good bacteria in your gut develop. Second and most importantly, you would need to restrain from all forms and kinds of sugar. Stop feeding the yeast to curb your cravings.

- *Adrenaline overload*

If you frequently suffer from bouts of hunger, irritability, sore throat, dizziness or stress, then you are undergoing an adrenaline overload. Other symptoms include being thirsty often and needing to urinate more frequently.

Adrenaline overload means that your adrenal glands are pumping out stress hormones namely cortisol and adrenaline when you are under pressure. If that constantly happens, the glands become lethargic or sluggish and you tend to crave for sugar to keep your energy up.

High-protein meals can provide you stable energy levels and diminishes your need for sugar. If your body has ample energy for the day, then you will be less stressed and the adrenal glands do not need to pump extra stress hormones to keep you up and going.

- *Menopause or PMT*

Women who have low moods, irregular periods and decreased sex drives are most probably experiencing menopause or perimenopause. Insomnia, fatigue, hot flushes and headaches are also symptoms of menopause or PMT.

This happens because progesterone and estrogen levels drop and women become prone to insulin sensitivity. Resistance to insulin can result to sugar cravings that, if not met, can cause irritability and fatigue. With the drop of female hormones, the body raises the levels of serotonin to make it feel good. This then triggers a sugar craving.

Taking Vitamin B6 will alleviate premenstrual tension and prostaglandin deficiency. Do not give in to sugar cravings during these moments as it will increase your tolerance for sugar. Cutting back will improve the production of prostaglandin that will make the body feel better and will significantly improve your mood.

Chapter 4: Blood Sugar Solutions

Blood sugar refers to the concentration or levels of glucose present in the body. Glucose is the fuel or energy source for the body's cells and systems. It is transported via the bloodstream and is absorbed by the cells with the help of insulin. Irregular blood sugar levels can cause fluctuations in insulin production. This may lead to grave diseases such as diabetes, kidney problems and heart problems, or even sugar addiction.

Do you know that you can curb your cravings? Here are some simple solutions you can easily adapt in your quest for a sugar-free life and establishing a good weight loss regimen.

Do not skip meals.

You need to eat regularly. When you body has enough fuel to burn for energy, you will keep your blood sugar stable. Hence, there will be no need for energy bursts that lead to sugar cravings or emotional eating behaviors. Be sure to fill up with foods that are rich in protein and fiber.

Distract yourself whenever you crave.

Get your mind on to other things and off that sugary stuff. Steer away from dessert tables at parties. Out of sight, out of mind is a good practice. If you do not have a cookie or doughnut staring you in your face, then it means you don't get to think about it. And before you even decide to open the fridge or go to the nearest coffee shop, then do something else like reading a book. Cravings will disappear when you don't attend to it. Let your mind dwell on other matters.

Take a drink when craving comes.

Whenever you feel the craving come in, take a glass of cold water. This will fill you up and satisfy you effectively, even if it is only temporary. You can vary your choice of beverage but refrain from taking sodas and fruit juices. Remind yourself that you are not succumbing to your craving.

Delay your gratification.

It means that you postpone giving in to your craving. Sometimes, giving yourself a few minutes of delay will make you lose the longing. For example, if you feel that you want that slice of triple chocolate cake, then put off eating it for about 30 minutes. Then eat half of it. Wait for another 30 minutes before you finish the other half. This will give you a sense of control over your desires and you will eventually have full control over your sugar cravings.

Think of how you can hate the very thing you love.

You love sweets and everything really looks nice and yummy. But if you really think about it, those things are just disgusting fats that can accumulate in your body. Think about the morbid effects it may have on your body. If you honestly view those things for what they really are, chances are you will not even go near them.

Move around!

Yes, instead of munching on that cookie or gulping down that soda, get your body moving. Dance, walk, do some jumping jacks, climb the stairs – anything that will not only keep your mind from eating sweets but also get your body to burn calories.

Try something new.

Go to the next chapters and see some exciting new recipes for smoothies and meals that you can make to help beat your sugar cravings.

Chapter 5: Sugar Addiction Detox Smoothies

When you are addicted to sugar, your body needs to undergo a detoxification process to flush out the unnecessary and unhealthy sugars within. A healthy and easy way to detoxify is to regularly drink smoothies.

Smoothies contain fruits and vegetables that are rich in fiber, minerals, vitamins and antioxidants. They promote weight loss and other health benefits associated with the fruit and vegetables that are incorporated in the beverage.

Fruits are naturally sweet but the potential harm of the sugar in fruits is not as weighty as the benefits they bring to the table. Fructose, or fruit sugar, is not the same as corn syrup or table sugar. It is a pure and concentrated sugar found in fresh, whole foods.

Here are some smoothies that you can whip up in your detoxification from sugar addiction.

Recipe 1:   COCONUT OIL SMOOTHIE

This is very nutritious, great tasting and will give you a boost of energy.

Ingredients

1 cup   apple

1 piece   ripe banana

1 ½ tablespoon virgin coconut oil

½ cup   yoghurt

1 cup   strawberries

3 cups   spinach

Directions

1.   Chop the apples into small pieces and put it in the blender with the yoghurt. Blend quickly, just enough to mix the yoghurt into the apples.

2.   Pour in the virgin coconut oil and whir until the VCO is blended throughout.

3.   Add the spinach, strawberries, and banana and blend until smooth. Enjoy your green smoothie!

Options to Coconut Oil Smoothie

You may opt to add protein powder (especially if you are going for a workout)

You can replace the yoghurt with water, kefir or coconut milk of you do not want dairy or are allergic.

Recipe 2:   BLUEBERRY-SPINACH SMOOTHIE

A healthy fiber, protein drink that will help keep your blood sugar steady and leave you feeling energized and craving-free.

Ingredients

1 cup	blueberries, frozen
1 cup	spinach
2 cups	coconut water
1 tbsp	chia seeds
1 tbsp	bee pollen
1 tbsp	hemp protein powder
1 tbsp	cacao
½ cup	ice cubes

Directions

1.   Combine coconut water blueberries, spinach, chia seeds, bee pollen and cacao in a blender and whir at high speed.

2.   Add in the hemp protein an blend quickly

3.   Put in the ice cubes and blend for another minute then you can enjoy your smoothie.

Recipe 3:   COFFEE-BANANA SMOOTHIE

A healthy alternative for coffee lovers!

Ingredients

1 piece	banana, ripened
1 cup	low-fat milk
½ cup	cold black coffee

2 pieces stevia leaves to sweeten

½ cup   ice cubes

Directions

1.   Combine all the ingredients and whir in a high-speed blender. Enjoy it cold!

Recipe 4:   BERRY FROSTY SMOOTHIE

Cool and refreshing smoothie for any kind of weather

Ingredients

1 cup   sugar-free lemon lime soda

2 pieces fresh mint leaves

½ cup   strawberry

1 cup   skim milk

1 cup   yoghurt

Directions

1.   Combine all the ingredients and whir in a high-speed blender. Enjoy your smoothie.

Recipe 5:   GRREN MOJITO SMOOTHIE

Healthy smoothie cocktail that can also be a remedy to colds and flu.

Ingredients

½ cup   pineapple

3 pieces fresh mint leaves

½ cup   kale

1 tsp   ginger

Directions

1.   Combine all the ingredients and whir in a high-speed blender. Enjoy your zesty smoothie.

Recipe 6:   THE GODDESS SMOOTHIE

Yummy smoothie fit for a queen.

Ingredients

3 cups   carrots, chopped

2 pieces large golden beets

3 pieces golden apples

½ cup   apricots (without pits)

Directions

1.   Combine all the ingredients and whir in a high-speed blender. Enjoy your smoothie.

You can mix your own favorite fruits and vegetables to make a great tasting detoxifying smoothie to cure your sugar addiction. Here are some important reminders to help you as you start making your healthy concoctions.

PROTEIN

Not every smoothie needs a protein. If you will use it as substitute for snack or an energy booster after workout, then you can add in some. Otherwise, enjoy it as a refreshing healthy drink that will flush out unwanted substances from your body.

In place of protein powders, you can use natural ingredients such as chia seeds, green yoghurt, egg whites, hemp seed and silken tofu.

SWEETENERS

Avoid using sugar or it will defeat the purpose of the smoothie. Use stevia, fenugreek and fruits to sweeten your smoothie naturally.

LIQUID

Coconut milk, soy milk, skim milk and regular low-fat milk are the common liquids used in preparing smoothies. You can add drops of vanilla for flavor. But remember that water is the best liquid ingredient, so if you can limit yourself to water, all the better for your health.

VEGETABLES

Greens such as kale, swiss chard and spinach mixed with the right fruits will give you the nutrients you need without the unfavorable taste. You can also use the following veggies for detoxification from sugar addiction: carrots, broccoli, zucchini and cucumber.

FRUITS

Almost any fruit will work with a smoothie but the best choices for beginners are bananas, pineapples, berries and oranges. The natural sweetness of the fruit masks the taste of the vegetables included, making it a more desirable drink.

OTHER HEALTHY ADD-ONS

Ground flaxseed is a high source of fiber and omega 3. Coconut oil is a source of good fat that can help curb sugar addiction.

Chapter 6: Sugar Detox Diet Recipe

If you are suffering from sugar addiction, you can undergo a 3-week detox challenge, wherein you will eat foods that will help cleanse your body and avoid certain foods such as processed sugars and grains.

Here is a guide:

Good Foods to Eat

(It is better if you can get them as organic produce)

Herbs

Vegetables, Except Potatoes

Avocado

Brown Rice

Carrots and Corn (Limit to ½ cup per serving)

Coconut Oil

Eggs

Fish

Goji Berries

Grape Seed Oil

Lemon and Lime

Nuts

Olive Oil

Organic Free-Range Meat Chicken and Turkey

Organic Grass-Fed Beef and Lamb

Quinoa

Sashimi

Tomatoes

Unsweetened chocolate

Wild Caught Salmon

Foods to Avoid:

Alcohol

Fried Foods

Artificial Sweeteners

Breads

Candy

Cereal

Cheese

Cream Sauces

Dairy

Flour

Fruit Juice

High Fructose Corn Syrup

Hydrogenated Oils

Maple Syrup

MSG: Monosodium Glutamate

Oatmeal

Potatoes

Raw Cane Sugar

Soy

Sugar

Trans Fats

Vinegar

Wheat Bread

White Rice

Yogurt

After the 3-week cleansing you can gradually add the following foods back to your diet: whole grains, fruits and natural sweeteners. However, processed grains and processed sugars are best avoided if you are to maintain a healthy body.

Some recipes you can try out during the 3-week detoxification are listed below:

Creamy Soup Recipe

Ingredients

1 head   celery

1 bunch asparagus

3 liters   chicken stock

1 large	onion
10 cloves	garlic
1 Tbsp	thyme
1 handful	parsley, chopped
1 teaspoon	coconut oil
2 cups	coconut milk or coconut cream

Ground pepper and salt to taste

Directions:

1. Prepare the ingredients by chopping the onions, garlic, asparagus, celery and zucchini and setting them aside.

2. Heat the coconut oil in a saucepot, then add onions and garlic. Stir fry until lightly browned.

3. Add the chopped asparagus, celery and zucchini and the chicken stock. Cover and let simmer for an hour.

4. Add the chopped parsley and simmer for another 5 minutes.

5. Remove from heat and puree in a blender until smooth.

6. Add in your cream and ground pepper and salt to taste.

7. Serve hot.

Roasted Bell Peppers & Cauliflowers Recipe

Ingredients

| 1 | red bell pepper, diced |
| 2 pounds | cauliflower, diced |

¼ cup	olive oil
1 ½ tsp	thyme
½ tsp	garlic
½ tsp	salt

Directions:

1. Preheat the oven to 400 degrees

2. Toss the diced cauliflower, diced bell peppers, thyme, garlic and salt with the olive oil in a large baking pan.

3. Bake for 30 minutes, uncovered.

4. Stir every 10 minutes and check for desired tenderness.

Ground Beef in Coconut Curry and Cabbage Bed Recipe

Ingredients

1 Tbsp	coconut oil
4 cloves	garlic, finely chopped
¼ cup	diced onion
1 cup	diced peppers
1 pound	beef (grass-fed)
1 teaspoon	salt
½ teaspoon	pepper
3 tsp	ground turmeric

1 teaspoon   cumin

1 teaspoon   ground coriander

1 Tbsp   curry powder

½ cup   tomato paste

1 can   coconut milk

½ inch   ginger, grated

½ teaspoon cayenne pepper (or dependent on your spice level)

   Juice from ½ lime

For the Steamed Cabbage:

1/2 head   cabbage

1 teaspoon   salt

Directions

1.   Before you begin cooking, be sure to measure out all of the spices and mix them all in a bowl. This will save you a lot of time and effort.

2.   Put coconut oil in a skillet and heat it to medium-high.

3.   Stir in the onions, garlic and sweet pepper making sure you coat them in coconut oil

4.   Add the ground beef and cook until browned through.

5.   Once the beef is cooked, add in the tomato paste.

6.   Grate some ginger right into the beef and paste mixture.

7.   Add all the spices you initially measured out and make sure everything is well mixed.

8.   Pour in the coconut milk and the lime juice and stir.

9. This dish is best served with on a plate of steamed cabbage (see recipe below) and topped with coconut curry.

Steamed Cabbage

1. Slice the cabbage and put it in a saucepan filled with 2 cups of water.

2. Cover the pan and put it on medium heat

3. Once it boils, turn the heat to low and let simmer for another 10 minutes

4. Toss the cabbage with salt and serve with the beef.

No Bake Healthy Fudge

Ingredients

1 cup	melted coconut butter
1 cup	pureed pumpkin
½ tsp	vanilla
4 Tbsp	cacao
3 Tbsp	coconut oil

Directions

1. Combine all ingredients in a food processor and mix until everything is fully blended.

2. Line up a pan with parchment or wax paper.

3. Scoop out the mixture into the pan.

4. Chill for four hours. Slice into desired pieces and enjoy.

Banana-Gelatin Pancakes

Ingredients:

2 pieces eggs

2 pieces bananas

1 Tbsp   gelatin

2 Tbsp   coconut oil

1 tsp   vanilla

Directions:

1.   Smash the bananas really well and whisk it in with the eggs.

2.   Add in the vanilla to taste and whist until there are no more lumps in the banana-egg batter.

3.   Pour in the gelatin

4.   Put coconut oil in a pan and heat it.

5.   When the coconut oil is ready, pour in small amounts of batter and allow the mixture to cook.

6.   When the sides are browned and crisp, which will take about 3 minutes, flip the pancake to cook the other side. It will take another 3 minutes.

Cauliflower Rice with Cilantro and Lime

Ingredients

1 head   cauliflower

1 bunch diced cilantro

1 tsp   cumin

Olive oil

Juice of 1 1/2 limes

Salt to taste

Directions

1.   Chop cauliflower florets, wash and leave to dry. When dry, put in processor and pulse until it is minced.

2.   Add oil to a heated skillet and put in the cauliflower. Cover and leave to cook for 5 minutes or until tender, while stirring occasionally.

3.   Remove from heat when cooked and add cilantro, lime juice, salt and cumin.

4.   Eat as a rice replacement.

Chapter 7: Use Of Coconut Oil To Cure Sugar Addiction

Coconut oil has a long list of health benefits and is a secret weapon to curbing cravings for sugar. For one, it makes you feel sated that you will surely have no appetite for sweets when you take a tablespoon or two of coconut oil after meals.

Coconut oil is consists of MCFAs or medium-chain fatty acids. MCFAs easily saturate cell membranes making them effectively utilized by the body. MCFAs put less strain on the digestive system because they are easily digested.

The body requires energy to move throughout the day and may encounter slumps in energy levels, which in turn produces the craving for sugar. The MCFA in coconut oil is a wonderful source of instant energy as it goes straight to the liver. Compared to carbohydrates that produce a spike in insulin levels, coconut oil delivers quick energy and saves you from an energy slump. No slump means no craving issues. Having no craving issues is a big step towards curing sugar addiction. Moreover, coconut oil is so filling that you will not be hungry for at least four hours.

Apart from curbing your cravings, coconut oil has other health benefits, too.

- *Coconut oil aids in weight loss*
  • The MCFAs in coconut oil becomes energy instead of being converted to fat. This happens as MCFAs go directly to the liver. Coconut oil likewise stimulates metabolism and increases thyroid activity, leading to loss of weight.

- *Coconut oil is anti-viral, anti-inflammatory and anti-fungal*

Coconut oil has rich lauric acid content. Lauric acid, found in breastmilk and coconut oil alone, is converted by the body to monolaurin. It is anti-bacterial, anti-protozoa and anti-viral. By increasing the body's metabolic rate, healing process speeds up and the immune system becomes healthier making the body less prone to inflammation.

- If you consider the many health benefits of using coconut oil and use it regularly, you are taking one big step on your way to curing your sugar addiction. You can add coconut oil to soups, stir-fries and smoothies.

Chapter 8: Natural Cinnamon And Honey To Cure Sugar Addiction

While honey is sweet, science says that it can be medicine when taken in the right doses. It actually is not a sugar threat and cannot harm even diabetics. Honey has potent enzymes that help cure many illnesses.

Natural cinnamon, on the other hand, is a spice bark that has bacteria-killing properties. Honey is 33 % organic sulfur based while cinnamon is 26%, making their combination a whopping 59% potent organic sulfur. Organic sulfur is a nutrient that is essential for the body but is not a prescription medicine or drug that can be obtained outside of nature. Sulfur increases the production of bodily enzymes which strengthens the immune system and the body's resistance to illness and disease.

Combining honey and cinnamon and taking it as a natural supplement and remedy gives therapeutic cure to the following:

- Heart disease
- Arthritis
- Upset stomach
- Bladder infections
- Colds
- Cholesterol
- Gas
- Influenza
- Skin infections
- Cancer
- Sore throat
- Toothaches

Honey and cinnamon combined will help curb sugar cravings for the following reasons:

1. It prevents fatigue.
   Put in a half tablespoon of honey and a sprinkle of cinnamon powder on a glass of water and take this as an elixir twice a day. This is proven to make the body more alert and lively. Fatigue and stress are often causes of sugar addiction.

2. It helps control blood pressure.
   Regular doses of cinnamon and honey will reduce high blood pressure and control insulin sensitivity. You can make cinnamon and honey spread for your daily bread intake.

3. It aids in digestion.
   Sprinkle natural cinnamon powder onto two tablespoons of honey. Eat this mixture before meals and you will find relief from acidity which results in good digestion. Proper digestion means that food is turned into the energy that your body needs and reduces your cravings for sugar.

4. The sulfur in cinnamon-honey mixtures reduces the risk of hypoglycemia or low blood sugar.

5. It helps improve PMS or PMT as it enhances production of glands. This diminishes the body's cravings for sugar associated with women's monthly periods.

Chapter 9: Guaranteed Herbal Remedies To Cure Sugar Addiction

The use of plants in improving health and treating diseases has been a widely accepted practice in the recent years. Medicinal herbs provide a natural and safer remedy to numerous common ailments, including sugar addiction.

The following herbal remedies curb sugar cravings with little to no side effects.

Stevia

Stevia is a plant whose leaves are naturally sweet that it is often called *sweet* leaf. Compared to regular sugar, it does not contain any calories but is a hundred times sweeter. Stevia increases the production of insulin and helps reduce blood sugar. This actually helps curb sugar cravings.

Instead of using sugar and other artificial sweeteners, use natural stevia leaves to sweeten your desserts and beverages.

Ginseng

Another popular herbal remedy is ginseng. It is a light-colored root herb that is shaped almost like a fork. Ginseng is a remedy to fatigue as it provides energy to the body and enhances well-being. Ginseng can also treat high levels of blood sugar.

When under a lot of stress, the body requires more energy to cope up with the conditions. Taking ginseng supplements regularly will sustain your energy levels, keep you from getting tired and help you avoid emotional eating and sugar cravings.

Fenugreek

Compared to stevia, fenugreek is mildly sweeter but its fragrance is the same as that of maple syrup. When you have sugar cravings, chewing on fenugreek leaves and seeds can help satisfy your sweet tooth. This herb helps control the fluctuations in the blood sugar. Regular use will cure sugar addiction.

Gymnema

A traditional herbal medicine that originated from India, gymnema sylvestre or gurmar can help stifle sugar addiction. Known in medical circles as the "sugar destroyer", chewing on gymnema leaves or sprinkling gymnena powder on the tongue suppresses taste buds' sweet receptors temporarily. You will then find sweet foods less pleasing and less satisfying. First, the mouth is filled with a sweet flavor, then the craving is conquered and you are left with a decreased response to sugar and little to no tendency of craving.

Gymnema also helps control insulin sensitivity and blood sugar levels.

These herbs are proven to help cure sugar addiction. But, like any health issue you may face, it is always best to consult with your physician or health care provider before you try it out.

It is important to remember not to self-diagnose, regardless of your health condition. If you are taking any specific medication or conventional drugs, do not stop it in favor of herbs without the approval your doctor. Herbal medicines are therapeutic and contain potent ingredients that should be treated with the same care and respect you would synthetic drugs.

Chapter 10: Responsible And Clean Eating To Cure Sugar Addiction

To break your sugar addiction, you need to start eating clean. Here are some actions you can take to ensure that you are taking care of your body and helping it work out its yearning for sugar.

1. Always hydrate. Drink eight to ten glasses of water a day (that is approximately 2 liters) to keep your body refreshed and feeling light. Sugar cravings are often a result of dehydration so when you feel a yearning for something sweet, drink a glass of water. To hydrate your system at the start of the day, take a smoothie for breakfast and drink a glass of water. Since smoothies contain highly digestible nutrients, your body is ready for hydration. Done regularly, this practice will curb your sugar cravings effectively.

2. Go for whole foods and low sugar diets. Make sure that your daily diet consists of whole foods that give your body the right amount of calories it needs. When you are low on calories, the body craves for sweet foods which are a quick source of energy. That is a primary reason why cookies, chocolates and other junk foods are popular afternoon snacks.

3. Whole foods like fish, vegetables, avocados, quinoa and grass-fed or fre range meats in your daily diet will cut your craving for sugars.

4. Refrain from artificial sweeteners and switch to natural sweeteners like stevia.

5. Take probiotics daily. These help restore balance to the digestive system and help your gut replenish intestinal flora or good bacteria. When our gut bacteria is out of balance, we

crave sugar. Probiotics help replenish intestinal flora and restore balance to the gut system. When the gut has a lot of bad bacteria, yeast and fungus, the body naturally craves sugar. Cut off the bad bacteria in your gut and you cut off your sugar cravings.

6. Topple the desire for sugar by eating the opposite of what you crave. Eat sour and fermented foods like kimchi and sauerkrauts whenever you want some sweets and you will find your natural desire slowly diminish. Moreover, these products contain probiotics and other essential nutrients.

7. Cut back on all simple sugars. Eat fruits instead of sweets.

8. Chew on find the some healthy, sugar-free gum to reduce your cravings.

9. Mix healthy foods with your sugar cravings. For example, dip a banana in chocolate syrup and you get the best of both worlds.

10. At times you can't help the craving and give in, remind yourself to eat just a little piece, to choose less sugary stuff and to eat it slowly.

> Oftentimes, denying your craving will cause you to want more, so give in just a wee bit. Choosing dark chocolate over a candy bar is a healthier sugar option. Eating slowly will cause your taste buds to savor the sweet and fill you up faster.

Remember that the human body is hypersensitive to sugar by nature. These strategies are doable as you work with your body. It may take a while but it is not an impossible task. Little steps that you incorporate in your life will amount to big amazing results in fighting off your sugar addiction.

Conclusion

Thank you again for purchasing this book on ULTIMATE SUGAR ADDICTION DETOX GUIDE: How To Beat Cravings Naturally and Cure Sugar Addiction With This Ultimate Sugar Detox Diet Formula!

I am extremely excited to pass this information along to you, and I am so happy that you now have read and can hopefully implement these strategies going forward.

I hope this book was able to help you understand sugar addiction and how to be free from its detrimental consequences.

The next step is to get started using this information and to hopefully live a healthier and happier life!

Please don't be someone who just reads this information and doesn't apply it, the strategies in this book will only benefit you if you use them!

If you know of anyone else that could benefit from the information presented here please inform them of this book.

Finally, if you enjoyed this book and feel it has added value to your life in any way, please take the time to share your thoughts and post a review on Amazon. It'd be greatly appreciated!

Thank you and good luck!

Preview Of:

<u>Sugar</u>

7 Day Sugar Junkie Detox Diet Plan To Beat Your Addiction And Rescue Yourself From Cravings Easily And Naturally With Clean Eating Recipes For Life!

Introduction

I want to thank you and congratulate you for purchasing the book, "Sugar: 7 Day Sugar Junkie Detox Diet Plan To Beat Your Addiction And Rescue Yourself From Cravings Easily And Naturally With Clean Eating Recipes For Life!"

This "Sugar" book contains proven steps and strategies on how to cut down your sugar intake in seven days without compromising your health.

This book includes:

- Recipes that will help reduce your consumption of sugar and carbohydrates.
- A simple 7-day meal plan that will help lower down your sugar cravings and help you lose weight.
- Helpful tips on how to stick on this detox and reap its maximum benefits.

The recipes contained in this book are also ideal for diabetics who wish to detoxify their body and reverse their Diabetes.

Whether you are suffering from diabetes or you are simple addicted to sugar and wants to live a healthier life, this book can help you achieve the healthier version of you.

Start flipping those pages and learn how to get in shape effectively.

Thanks again for purchasing this book, I hope you enjoy it!

Chapter 1: What Is Sugar Addiction?

Sugar addiction is the dependence on sugar consumption. People who are addicted to sugar commonly eat more than they intend to, they crave for sugar and they lose control. Sugar addicts can't stop eating sweet treats such as cakes, pastries, soda and other carbohydrates-filled foods and products.

According to experts, eating sugar causes the brain to release more Dopamine, which is a neurotransmitter that plays a major role in a person's emotions, sense of pleasure and pain, drive and desire to get things done. When we eat sugary foods in large amounts, it causes the Dopamine receptors to downgrade. Therefore, there are fewer receptors for Dopamine. When this happens, the next time we consume foods that have high sugar content the effect is considerably weaker than before; which is why we need to eat more to get the same feeling.

Due to the effects of sugar to the rewards center of the brain, sugar addiction functions the same as drug abuse such as nicotine and cocaine. Just like drug addiction, people get addicted to sugar and lose control over their consumption. This is basically how sugar affects the brain so that we crave for more and eat more.

Sugar addiction can lead to a myriad of health issues such as heart diseases, binge eating, cravings and weight gain. Research also shows that a diet rich in sugar increases the risk for Type II Diabetes, causes significant decrease in HDL (good) cholesterol and elevated triglycerides. Too much sugar intake is also linked to migraine, depression, poor eyesight, gout, osteoporosis and autoimmune diseases such as multiple sclerosis and arthritis.

The more sugar we consume, the more tolerant we become. Our strong craving for sugar is not because of our genes. It is actually due to our food choices and dietary habits. This means you can reverse the effects of sugar addiction. Sugar Detox Diet is an effective way of cutting down on sugar consumption. Once you have undergone a Sugar Detox Diet, you will no longer have cravings for sweet treats and you will start eating better.

Thanks for Previewing My Exciting Book Entitled:

"Sugar: 7 Day Sugar Junkie Detox Diet Plan To Beat Your Addiction And Rescue Yourself From Cravings Easily And Naturally With Clean Eating Recipes For Life!"

To purchase this book, simply go to the Amazon Kindle store and simply search:

"SUGAR"

Then just scroll down until you see my book. You will know it is mine because you will see my name "Sarah Brooks" underneath the title.

Alternatively, you can visit my author page on Amazon to see this book and other work I have done. Thanks so much, and please don't forget your free bonuses

DON'T LEAVE YET! - CHECK OUT YOUR FREE BONUSES BELOW!

Free Bonus Offer: Get Free Access To The www.LiveFitVIP.com VIP Newsletter!

Once you enter your email address you will immediately get free access to this awesome newsletter!

But wait, right now if you join now for free you will also get free access to the "The 7 Keys To Body Transformation" free EBook!

To claim both your FREE VIP NEWSLETTER MEMBERSHIP and your FREE BONUS Ebook on THE 7 KEYS TO BODY TRANSFORMATION!

Just Go To:

www.liveFitVIP.com

www.ingramcontent.com/pod-product-compliance
Lightning Source LLC
Chambersburg PA
CBHW071146280526
45787CB00003B/1425